Psychology Of Success

How to Succeed When Trying to
Change How You Look

Joyce Zborower, M.A.

ISBN-10: 1481208519
ISBN-13: 978-1481208512

DEDICATION

Changing your body image may be the hardest thing any of us have ever tried to do. This book provides extensive documented research into what it takes to have success when trying to change how you look. I dedicate this work to everyone who has ever tried and failed – and tried again ... including me.

Table of Contents

Prologue

His name was Jim Robinson. Like many fat gainers, past 30, he was struggling to lose weight. He was willing to try anything. His ever expanding waistline made Jim desperate to try anything that might help.

Ironically, in his younger days, Jim was self-consciously thin. Exercise didn't interest him, though he played the odd basketball game, with friends. Jim did not smoke. He enjoyed the occasional beer, but never drank to excess.

Jim's body structure changed, for the worse, when he entered his twenties. He developed an excessive fondness for beer and food.

Professionally, Jim did well. He became a purser, with a domestic airline. The job paid reasonably, and Jim married Jenny, his sweetheart of many years. Jenny worked as a secretary, in a law firm. The good times looked like they were lasting forever.

And suddenly, there was trouble in paradise...

To an extent, Jim's problems could be ascribed to the nature of his job. He was flying most days of the month. When he wasn't flying, he was at home - for days, at a stretch. Jim would be alone, at home, while Jenny was at work. Jim soon acquired another compelling interest to add to beer and food – TV! Jim became the quintessential couch potato.

The airline Jim worked for sacked him . . . for carrying excess baggage. His uniform shirts didn't fit any longer. Things got even worse. Jenny lost her job, too, when the law firm she worked in filed for bankruptcy. . .

Introduction

The Battle of Waterloo was won on the playing fields of Eton. Likewise, your battle against weight gain is actually won - or lost - in your mind. Your thoughts guide your actions: a motivated and determined mind is what you will need most, when you buckle down to getting a better looking body.

Making up your mind is not easy; harder still, is maintaining your resolve in the face of the challenges you are likely to face, as you strive to convert thought into action. Many like you have tried and failed. A few have succeeded, and succeeded well. You would surely want to be counted among the winners, wouldn't you?

So, how do you succeed in your effort to slim down and look sexy and attractive? Or more precisely, what kind of mental makeup do you need in order to succeed? Once you have a game plan in place, what does it take for you to stick to your resolve?

In this report, I take a deeper look at the problem, and lay bare the secrets of winners – those who have found the solution!

Begin By Identifying the Problem

While most people want to look great, they balk at the thought of having to do difficult exercises. This gradually weakens their resolve to look attractive. Eventually, they give it up altogether.

Looking great does not mean looking like a glamorous model on TV or being muscular like a professional body-builder. An attractive body need not always be muscular. Merely having a flat tummy could draw a comment such as: "Hey Jim, you look great, how did you do it?" I presume you aspire to be like *this* "Jim". This is an eminently achievable goal. But most of those who aspire to it never actually get there . . . either because they are either unwilling to start or, if they have begun the journey, are unwilling to continue, for some perceived reason or another.

Could this be why most people in America are either overweight or obese?

By 2000, there were about 127 million Americans who were overweight while there were nearly 60 million people who were obese and about 9 million who were very obese. (Source: http://obesity1.tempdomainname.com/subs/fastfacts/obesity_US.shtml).

But the latest survey reports from NIDDK show that more than 60% of American adults who are above 20 years are overweight. (Source: http://www.wrongdiagnosis.com/artic/understanding_adult_obesity_niddk.htm).

Some CDC (Center for Disease Control) reports from survey data suggest that more than half of American adults (above 57%) are overweight. This percentage translates to nearly 39.8 million American adults. (Source: http://www.wrongdiagnosis.com/o/obesity/basics.htm).

But if you don't want to be the "Jim" of my first paragraph, you need to take some urgent steps to get into shape. This is likely to take time as it involves more than just wishful thinking. You have to work, and work *hard*. And that requires that you stay determined and keep reminding yourself about your objective, until you reach the moment of truth when you can shout out, "I did it! I have done what I set out to do."

Ask any successful LOSER (weight loser) how he did it and his answer is almost always going to be, "I stuck with my resolve. I worked hard and now I have got it." If they can, so can you.

There are several examples of how people have tried and achieved the results they desired. And they are not necessarily athletes, but many of them are ordinary people.

Sports professionals who become obese need to regain fitness and shape, in order to remain competitive. They sometimes get support. But ordinary people do not have any such support. Yet, many have succeeded. There are many such success stories you can read about, here: http://www.nwcr.ws/stories.htm).

Preparing To Fight the Problem

Fighting excessive weight gain or obesity is never going to be easy, but you can achieve it if you are following a scientific step-by-step approach:

- **Motivating Yourself**

Motivation is the key. Embarking on your journey without motivation is like attempting to cut down a giant oak by using a blunt ax. Professional sports persons train hard all year round; they are driven by the conviction that, in the end, they will taste success. The motivation to succeed is essential to their dream of achieving the success and glory that other professionals achieve -- and that they envy. And it often takes them several months, and sometimes even years, of patient hard work, to get there.

You don't necessarily have to be built like an athlete to be considered good looking. A slim body with sexy flat abs is enough to make you feel great and achieve the same kind of recognition from people who matter to you -- friends, companions, and others around you. You want them to look admiringly at you, and say, "Hey Jim, you look great!"

Sports persons look forward to a long, successful and financially rewarding career. That desire keeps them motivated. As long as they stay focused on their goal, they remain on track. But other men and woman have other reasons to reduce weight or, to be exact, acquire a slim waist. Different ordinary people have different motivations.

Carolyn weighed 252 pounds when she suddenly lost her husband. Determined not to go her husband's way, she adopted sensible eating habits and a more active lifestyle. Carolyn is now down to 150 pounds and looks and feels great.

Or, take the case of Gary Pierce. Like Carolyn, a personal tragedy motivated him. Not only did he manage to check his weight, his efforts also helped him overcome his tragedy. (Read his real life story here: http://www.nwcr.ws/stories.htm). Now, past age 40, he is a real life example of my mythical "Jim".

- **Transforming Motivation into Action**

Having begun, it is easy to give up quickly when you don't see the results you expected. Most people are irritated by the difficulties they face when following a routine. Their determination falters; they look for excuses to give up. Once escapist tendencies set in, the battle is all but lost. Ask most people who've failed, and they will recite a story with several reasons for quitting. They lost the battle in their minds first . . . then they gave up.

When you start putting into practice what you have planned, you are certain to make some mistakes. You could easily get disheartened with no results. Often, people can be heard complaining, "I have been doing this for weeks now, but the result is zero – zilch -- nada". It takes time and effort to burn fat. Even when you use the right approach, your body will take time to burn fat. You just have to keep trying harder and analyze your actions. Only those who have stuck with their resolve and continued to work against despair have succeeded. In the example above, Gary Pierce succeeded because he kept trying. He concentrated on his body, and did not worry about anything else.

Another mistake that most people commit is in trying to be perfect. You have to remember not to aim for perfection immediately on beginning a program. Only with practice will you be able to do something perfectly. That requires you to determinedly follow the regime you have planned for yourself.

There is always the danger that you will make mistakes and feel guilty. The guilt feeling could introduce negatives in your mind. To counter this, you need to do things slowly. Gradual progress can give lasting results. Learning to enjoy your workouts is one way to counter the negatives cropping up in your mind. Many successful sports persons have achieved this.

In fact, the psychologists working with the American Board of Sports Psychologists, who counsel sports professionals, are often known to say that they guide their clients by encouraging them to adopt long term strategies; This is the preferred approach, rather than providing them with immediate short term solutions when their clients find it difficult to handle stress.

The stress can be in the form of physical stress (symptom: tiredness, fatigue) and/or mental stress (wanting to stop, or give up). They argue against adopting instant results solutions as this is only likely to harm the body over a period of time. The psychologists support a prolonged and controlled approach towards maintaining fitness. You can choose a similar pattern, for your program. Aim for long a longer duration of workouts spread over months, instead of days or weeks, or a quick results approach. Only this will help you overcome your negative emotions whenever you face them.

You would be amazed at how many people quit easily when faced with pressure. Take a look at the statistics provided at - http://answers.google.com/answers/threadview/id/138544.ht ml Here is some interesting information from that page:

At the website, http://www.dovico.com/time-management-factsandfigures.html,
Dr. Donald E. Wetmore says that about 90 out of a hundred people who join gyms for the purpose of exercising often quit within 90 days of joining.

Similar statistics are given at
http://www.healthandfitness.com/resources/gym_evaluation .asp
stateing that, of all those who join gyms for workouts, nearly 40 % will stop using their membership. However, a fifth of the members regularly make good use of their membership by exercising at the gyms. They are determined to workout no matter what hardships they face. It is this category of people you should aim to belong to.

Here's a graphical representation that shows how many people join gyms following a new year's resolution:

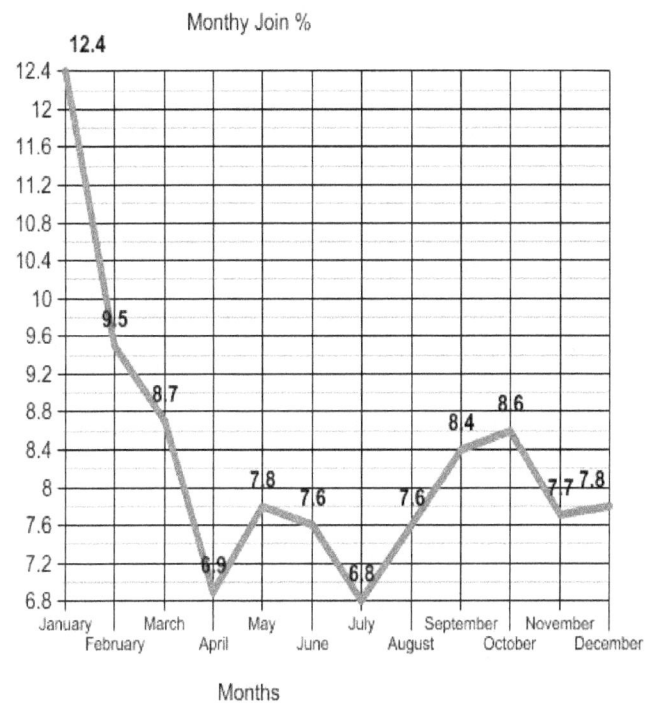

Monthy Join %

Months

http://www.ihrsa.org/industrystats/add.html

Stop Procrastinating – Act Now

Once you have planned to exercise, get on with it as soon as you can, or else you may never be able to take the first step. Most people either aren't brave enough to take the plunge, or if they do take the plunge, look for ways to get out. Putting it off for tomorrow is not going to help you in any way. Rather, you are delaying taking corrective measures by one more day and you are also then closer to bad health and problems . . . by a day. You should aim to achieve good health, a great looking body and confidence, which you will only get once you take action.

Overcoming your inhibitions requires a strong will. It is with this will that you resolved to have a flat abdomen, now it's time to prove to yourself that you are really that strong. I say "to yourself" because it's your abdomen, and no one else can flatten your abs for you.

Excuses You Should Avoid

You will often be faced with problems such as strenuous workouts, laziness and an inclination to simply stop. But you have to learn to avoid these excuses if you want to be a real life hero, like Gary Pierce. You don't always have to aim for that muscular look like the models you see on TV or in glossy magazines. Just having a flat tummy along with a fit body is what you should aim for. In fact, even if you do achieve a very muscular physique like a bodybuilder's, you will find it very hard to maintain that look for long. You don't want to look like you are all brawn and no brain. You can certainly do better looking smart and sexy. This is also easier to maintain over a lifetime.

But to get there you need to learn to overcome your excuses. Here are some of the most commonly offered excuses by people whose resolve is beginning to falter:

- "I don't have the time to exercise."

How many of us have the time to exercise when there are so many things to be done? But if you want to have an attractive/ healthy body, then you need to find the time. It's through exercise proper eating that you can get the shape you want. You can't just buy a good looking body for yourself, nor can you get that look just by wishing for it. This is almost the first thing you will hear from a person not wanting to take that plunge, or who just wants to quit. You will probably hear this from those 90% of the people who quit within the first three months of joining a gym.

- "I don't think I am overweight now, so I can wait and watch."

Is this really what you want to believe? If so, you have been playing with yourself, all this while. You know clearly that once the urge is lost, it's difficult to get it back. You have to hold on to it. But now, you are letting yourself lose that grip. Don't ever forget what you aimed for when you started out. Are you really there, or is there still a long way to go? Almost everybody will have a negative answer to this question. Not bothering about maintaining their looks once they have achieved it is a common phenomenon, especially among men.

- Dieting can provide equally good results.

This is a myth. Dieting alone won't do it for you. Anyway, how long can you maintain a diet? And what about those days when you have to work on an empty stomach. Doesn't your body crave food during that time? And how do you compensate for being hungry then? By eating whatever you can lay your hands on. And there go; all your diet plans out the window!

This is the pattern of what's called 'yo-yo' dieting. What you need is balanced food intake, meaning, a few calories, proteins and fiber, served with a bit of exercise. The last item is important as only this will actually build the muscle that you can't get with a diet.

- "I feel shy when I see so many fit bodies at the gym." Yes, there will be a lot of good looking men and possibly women, too, at the gym. But it's possible that they all came there with unfit bodies, and, in all probability, potbellies. They have their current shape because they practiced what they believed. They have actually translated their desires into actions and are enjoying the results in the form of a shapely and sexy looking body now. So can you.

- "It's all too expensive." All gym memberships are expensive. But when you joined, you didn't bother about expense. You just wanted a good looking body. Why has this sudden thought of expense crept into your mind, now? Can't you really afford to use a gym, or exercise equipment? . . . or have your priorities changed? Whatever it may be, you should not ignore the need to exercise to maintain shape.

- "I can jog -- that will reduce weight."

Activities like jogging, cycling, swimming do help reduce weight. But if you want to flatten your tummy then you need strong ab muscles to hold it in that shape. These can only be developed by exercising those muscles. Jogging may not be tiresome for many, but exercising the muscles will certainly be tiring. And that is the reason people tend to look for excuses. Always remember that you will have a good looking abdomen only when your ab muscles have been strengthened. You either exercise to get what you want, or forget about owning a good looking waist.

- "Exercise isn't the only way to good health."
Admittedly, exercise alone is not the solution. But exercise keeps at bay problems that can make you feel incapacitated in real life. You need vigor and fitness, but what can really make you feel confident is the good looks (that others admire and envy) that you will get only with exercise. In no other way can you get into shape nearly as fast.

- "Isn't there a pill that can replace exercise?"
Couldn't we all use such a pill! If pills could do everything, then why would we even bother to eat? Dreaming of pills to replace your physical activity is akin to seeking a short-cut past your problems. You know, as well as everyone else does, that there can be no shortcuts if you want a sexy looking tummy or if you want to hear people telling you that you look great.

- "I can do it tomorrow."
That's procrastination at work in your mind . . . And wishful thinking, too. This is how you could move away from exercising. And once you have done that it's going to be very difficult to come back to the first stage.

It's probably fatigue or boredom to blame . . . Your mind is beginning to waver; now is when you need to hold on to your dream tightly because if you let it slip now, things will only get worse with every passing day. Then, it's all a waste of effort, and time. You have resolved to have a good looking body, and that resolve is weakening. There will be many more such occasions that will test your resolve. Take these as periodic tests that you must pass to go on to the next level and get closer to your goal.

- "I can't go on. I give up. I will try again . . . some other time."

This is a sign that the final link between your resolve and your goal is breaking. Once you allow this thought to enter your mind, every time you start exercising, you would be inventing an excuse beforehand for failure. And each time you try to restart, you will be reminded of past failures. Those thoughts will play in your mind, repeatedly, and it will take a long time to overcome this pattern. You will need a will of steel to do so. By focusing on your final aim, you can prevent any weakening of your resolve.

- "I will never lose weight."

There can be many reasons for this kind of defeatist thinking. If this is what you think even before you have started exercising, you are probably trying to avoid physical work. Another reason you think this way could be that even after exercising for weeks or months, you don't see any difference. This could be either because you did not follow the correct exercise techniques or you were expecting quick results where none was forthcoming. Either way, you are putting too much pressure on yourself, and that is sure to hurt you.

How You Can Avoid Excuses

You have to encourage yourself; don't rely on someone else to motivate you. You must accept that to succeed in any effort, you have to sacrifice something. Follow a scheduled weight loss program. A schedule guides you and helps you understand your progress through regular reports you can prepare about yourself. You also have to check to see if you are expecting results to appear too soon. What is the period of time you have set yourself for weight loss? Are you aiming at overall improvement in health with looking good as a bonus or are you just trying to look attractive? You are more likely to succeed if you adopt the first objective.

I have only mentioned a few of the excuses people resort to, in order to avoid exercise. The International Health, Racquet and Sports club Association (IHRSA) is a non profit organization that provides assistance to people to change their lifestyles for the better. IHRSA has done a study of how and why people quit after taking up some form of exercise, and they have displayed the results on their website. Take a look at what they are, here:

http://cms.ihrsa.org/index.cfm?fuseaction=page.viewPage&pageID=20876

Remind yourself every now and then about what you have set out to do. This will allow you to judge how far you have come. For example, when you are fresh in the morning, remind yourself that you have to exercise today. Then make sure you find time for exercise during the day or at the allotted time. Before you retire for the day, ask yourself, "Have I exercised today? How much did I workout today? What difference has that made to my body?" With regular exercise, you will be able to answer these questions easily, daily. The greater ease and freedom you answer these questions with, the greater you'll build up your confidence. You will notice the results, physically, when you see your waist size shaping into what you want it to be.

Setting Realistic Goals

This is as important a part of the the program as your resolve. It's importance lies in the fact that you can only set the right goals once you have understood what you really want, what you are capable of doing, what you are willing to do to achieve the goal and how strong you will be when under pressure to quit. Setting yourself a target waist size is the first step. Planning how to get it is the next step. When you actually start working, you will encounter difficulties you had not thought of, or not planned for. What, then?

If, for instance, you have set yourself a target waist size of 32 or 34 inches, to be achieved over a period of six months, and at the end of the fifth month you find that you are nowhere near your target, you could panic. This could result in confusion, and in turn, lead to one wrong decision after another. If you notice that you are lagging behind, then you need to look back and analyze where you erred. But you need not stop your exercise regime. Doing that could make you slip back further and undo all the good work you have already done. Once you have zeroed in on your errors, aim to correct those in the next six month schedule you will start immediately after the current schedule is over.

Setting a long term goal and trying to reach it can become a burden. If it seems like an unachievable mirage, try establishing short term goals that will ultimately lead to achieving your final objective. Achieving such short term objectives is easier and these positives could encourage you into believing that you are capable of meeting the long term objectives you have set for yourself.

Bracing Yourself for the Task Ahead

Determination is a basic necessity when setting out to achieve something. In your case you want to get a flat tummy and look sexy. You could get slim in many ways, but how badly do you want to? To be able to realize your desire, you need to act. But there's no magic wand that'll help you achieve the healthy mental attitude you need to face the challenge:

1. Avoiding Negative Influences And Unsolicited Advice

You have to plan your exercise program according to *your* body. If you start on a highly enthusiastic note after being prompted from someone else to do so, then you are probably not setting your goal based on your own understanding of your body, but on others' perception. You are the best judge of your own body. If you have any difficulty with this, consult a gym instructor where you exercise, or get some professional advice. They can prepare a plan for you and offer consultative advice based on what type of plan you want to follow. Once you have chosen and started working on the plan do not allow a stray remark to disturb you, or a passing comment to derail your effort. Understand that it will take time, and you will win, ultimately.

Avoiding negative remarks or comments is a way of guaranteeing success. This will test your resolve. How well you maintain yourself under such pressure will be a test of the strength of your mind. But why waste energy and time on that when all you want is good looks that will attract positive and well meaning comments from others, like "Hey Jim, you look great".

2. Changing Habits, When Habits Die Hard

Habits are always difficult to change. Our mental make up plays an important part in how strongly we hold on to our habits. But if these habits come in the way of your objective then they have to go, too. Getting rid of the habits that act as obstacles in your path to a shapely waist is crucial to your success. And unless you are willing to give up some of your old habits for a larger goal or towards a good looking body, you will always find that target slipping away even when it's within reach.

Changing habits is easier said than done. Acknowledging your negative habits is only the first step. Overcoming them is the next and more important step. Small things can make a difference, such as foregoing an after meal sweet or slouching on a sofa or munching on something as you watch TV. Foregoing a snack at the office or even avoiding driving to the supermarket a few streets away can be things that could make a big difference in how quickly you reach your target. Your goal calls for such simple sacrifices, so you are sure of reaping the rewards later.

3. Guarding Against Mood Swings, Depression And Euphoria

One reason why many young people in America are obese is because they find it difficult to control their moods. Most people try to compensate for emotional upheavals or depression by overeating. They find solace in food. Eating improperly under such stressed conditions isn't going to help you at all. A large percentage of the population in the US is overweight because they do not eat properly, or tend to eat when stressed.

If you find yourself succumbing to an uncontrolled feeding problem, then consider this, for example. Even when you are depressed, or when you are under extreme stress, you don't stop earning, or give up your livelihood. Similarly, if you notice that you are struggling to control your food intake, remind yourself that losing weight and gaining a great shape is a goal you have set for yourself, and you should not falter.

Enjoying good food is alright, but splurging on food should not become a way of diverting attention from your problems. Just like you resolved to lose weight to look attractive, similarly, learn to combat the thoughts that could become hindrances.

At the same time, it is necessary to keep tabs on your behavior. Just like mood swings can cause you to lose or gain weight, your behavioral patterns can also influence your objectives. Under a perceived or actual stimulus you could unwittingly change your pattern of exercise that could disrupt your scheduled steps towards successful completion of the program. This has been proven through a test conducted by professionals by JAMA (The Journal of American Medical Association). Their studies have shown a direct link between behavioral patterns with weight loss and an improved appearance of the body in a group of people who were being monitored. The group being studied for behavioral patterns was able to achieve a reduction in their waist sizes slightly faster than those who did not receive any therapy. The results of the study should be of interest to anybody who has realized the benefit of changing their behavior for good. You can see the test results for yourself, here:

http://jama.ama-assn.org/cgi/content/abstract/285/9/1172

4. Visualizing Yourself In The Form You Desire

Imagining how you will look in a few months from now, in that shape, in those clothes, and in the company you desire, should keep you excited. However, don't get disheartened if it takes time. People often feel discouraged when they don't see the results they expected to see within a predetermined time. Realizing your hopes and aspirations takes time, whether it's your life's ambition, or something as simple as getting sexy looking abs. When you can and have overcome so many difficult situations, thus far, getting into shape should be something not so hard to achieve. If you have been successful, so far, it's because you have set success, in whatever you set out to do, as your priority. Now, you just have to set your priority to achieving that flat tummy.

Visualizing yourself in whatever shape you want to be, in some time from now, and refreshing that memory every time you exercise, is one way to keep yourself motivated. Do this, and you will find yourself working harder and with greater determination.

Most people visualize themselves as being slim and attractive, in the future. That is why they spend so much money on attaining the shape they have visualized themselves in. It is not for nothing that Americans have spent nearly $60 billion on buying equipment to get into shape See the FDA report, and the results of the search done by the firm Marketdata, here:
http://www.worldometers.info/weight-loss/

A point that should be of interest to many overweight and fat people who would like to reduce their weight quickly is that when we reduce our weight quickly, there is no time left for the skin to contract back into shape. The result is that though we may have burned the extra stored fat, we will still look slightly fat with hanging skin seen in folds. This could be much uglier than just looking fat. This is another reason why it is preferable to lose weight slowly.

5. Comparing What You Have Gained, When You Look Back

Weight reduction and a great body shape can't be got just by wishful thinking. Quick fixes do not work with weight reduction. Tiredness, fatigue and frustration will compel you to look back. You could find it difficult to control your wavering mind. You will frequently be tempted to think back on the days since you started exercising. And the end results are not going to be what you expected. You will understand this to be a common complaint among weight reduction enthusiasts when you discuss your progress in a group. So what do you do?

Try to compare what you have gained and what you have lost. That waist of yours may not have decreased as much as you would have expected it to, but you feel fitter now, don't you? You have more stamina, can work longer without getting tired and you certainly feel more flexibility in your body than before. Isn't that a gain? Becoming more flexible is an achievement that comes only when you are fit and when you are in shape. This is an indication that you are on your way to sliming your waist, and getting an attractive body. Reminiscences of the past (your failures) will always spring up at the most unexpected moment. But with a thought concentrated on the future rewards, you will gradually learn to overcome these moments.

6. Understanding The Desire To Fit In

Nowadays many want to be thin because it's fashionable, and because we are influenced a lot by what we see around ourselves. We feel good and comfortable blending in and being accepted. But that should not be the primary reason you want to look great. You have to look forward to an improved lifestyle as the real benefit. Being accepted will come as a bonus, automatically.

If your weight control program or the reason you chose to flatten your tummy is only the desire to look great, you might aim for quick results that you are unlikely to get. Even if you did manage to drastically alter your appearance, you would have problems maintaining the results.

You need to set a healthy life as your ultimate aim else all your efforts are likely to be short-lived, doing more harm than good.

A survey conducted by the American Time Use Survey during the 2003 - 2006 time period showed that people who have had higher education are the ones that are more likely to exercise. The study also found that people above 25 years of age possessing a bachelor's degree were the most open to exercising. Take a look at the findings, here:
http://www.bls.gov/spotlight/2008/sports/data.htm#chart02

Here's a graphical representation of the findings:

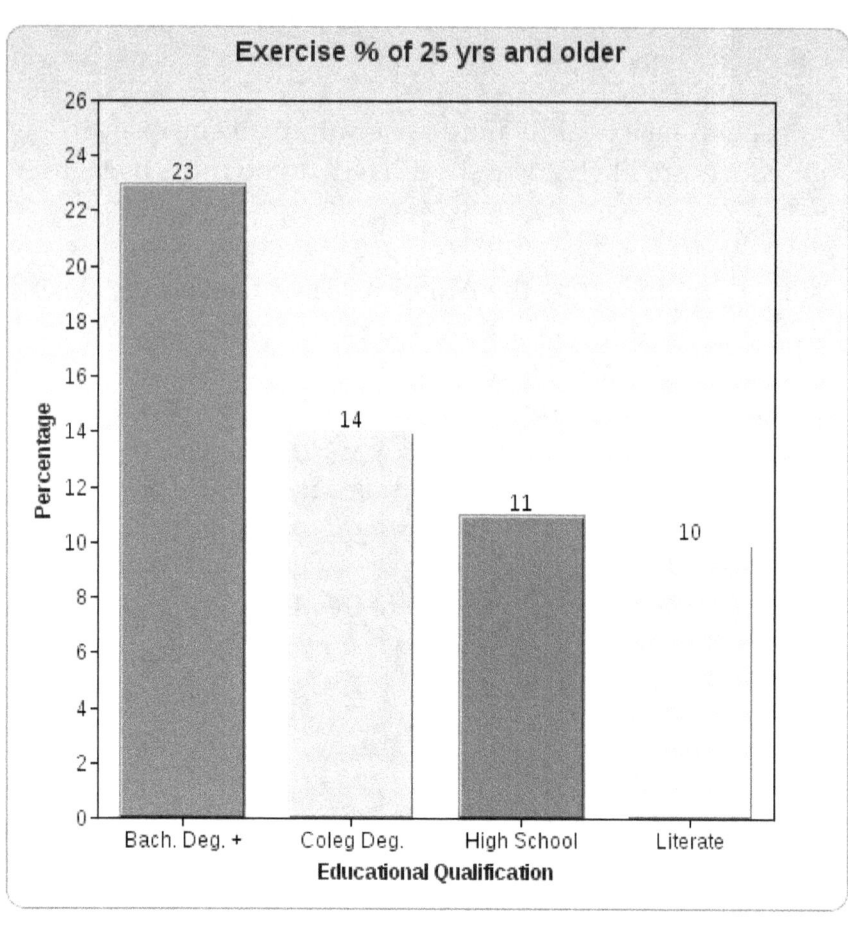

Re-building Your Mental Makeup – And Your Body

You need determination to be able to reduce weight. And afterwards, there will be a lot of hard work, as well. Till now, you have probably accepted the way you look. But now, you have an urge to reduce your weight and look better. Therefore, you need to recast or mold yourself in the way you desire.

-Your Body Image

What you think of your body plays an important part in deciding how you are going to act to improve it. Your opinion about yourself - physically and emotionally - will affect your behavior, and this, in turn, will judge what you plan to do, and how you plan to do it.

According to a survey conducted by CDC (Center for Disease Control) nearly 67% of the adult population is overweight. (See here - http://www.news-medical.net/news/20090904/Americans-health-perceptions-contradict-national-statistics.aspx)

But only 25 % of the people actually think they are overweight. As you can see, there is hesitation to admit to being overweight. On the other hand, there may be some who are anorexic and consider themselves overweight, when, in fact, they are not.

In a similar survey by Mintel, 70% of the respondents replied that they thought they needed more exercise. On being asked how much they exercised, only 37% said they were regular, while nearly half the respondents said that they exercised two days in a week, or fewer. So, you can see how lot of people are able to convince themselves, based on what they want to believe, or what kind of activity they are willing to undertake. Compare this with the statistics of CDC and you will see a great difference. And nearly half of those questioned, about 51% , replied that they give preference to a healthy lifestyle.

This is just an example of how people's opinion about themselves can influence their actions.

In another study done by Weight-control Information Network (WIN), a group under the National Institute of the Diabetes and Digestive and Kidney Diseases (NIDDK), it was revealed that almost half the adult population used some form of vigorous physical exercise to maintain fitness, and about one quarter of the population did not use any form of physical activity to maintain their bodies. Look here for the reference: http://www.win.niddk.nih.gov/statistics/index.htm#other

- Self Monitoring

It could be as simple as noting down your weight, every weekend, as an index of your progress. Or it can contain complex procedures that can mean you noting down the mood you were in before and after the exercise, the food you ate, the duration for which you exercised, the number of days you exercised in a week, the types of exercises you tried, etc.

Many health professionals agree that self monitoring of the progress made in weight control is an important step towards the realization of this goal. How this affects your mental make up can be gauged by how encouraged or discouraged you feel when you see your weight change, or when there is no change at all. Such monitoring not only warns you of an unnatural weight gain, it gives you a feeling of having gone one step closer to your goal. But frequently checking your weight - sometimes more than once daily -- can signal a hidden discomfort, which is expressing itself in this form of frenzied weight checks. When you notice yourself doing this, you need to understand your condition. This can also indicate other disorders, possibly related to depression. Do not let such tendencies spoil an otherwise natural progression into a healthy lifestyle. In fact, this can also indicate a behavioral abnormality that you also need to check, because that is another factor that can lead to variations in weight.

Self monitoring can have a positive, or negative, effect on your mind. You must learn to set aside all the negative and try to focus on what you want to achieve in order to get there.

- Congratulating Yourself On Battles Won

There is nothing wrong in congratulating yourself on victorious battles, no matter how small they may seem. Tomorrow, you will cherish these memories. After this, whenever you look back, these will stand out as strong indicators of your achievements. No one else can do this for you, and probably no one else will understand this as well as you can. It's important to you and that is what ultimately matters, for your confidence.

Overcoming Faulty Thoughts Regarding Your Body

Most of us, when we evaluate ourselves, tend to be harsh, in our judgment. This is also influenced by what we see, when we compare ourselves with others, who are better looking than us. This often raises a tendency to be perfect in our physical appearance. There is also a need to control such perfectionist tendencies. If you succumb to such tendencies then you are putting unnecessary pressure on yourself which will affect your weight loss program adversely.

To find out what percentage of people think they weigh more than normal when they are actually so, take a look at the chart at the following link:
http://www.infoplease.com/ipa/A0763634.html

Here is a graphical representation of the data.

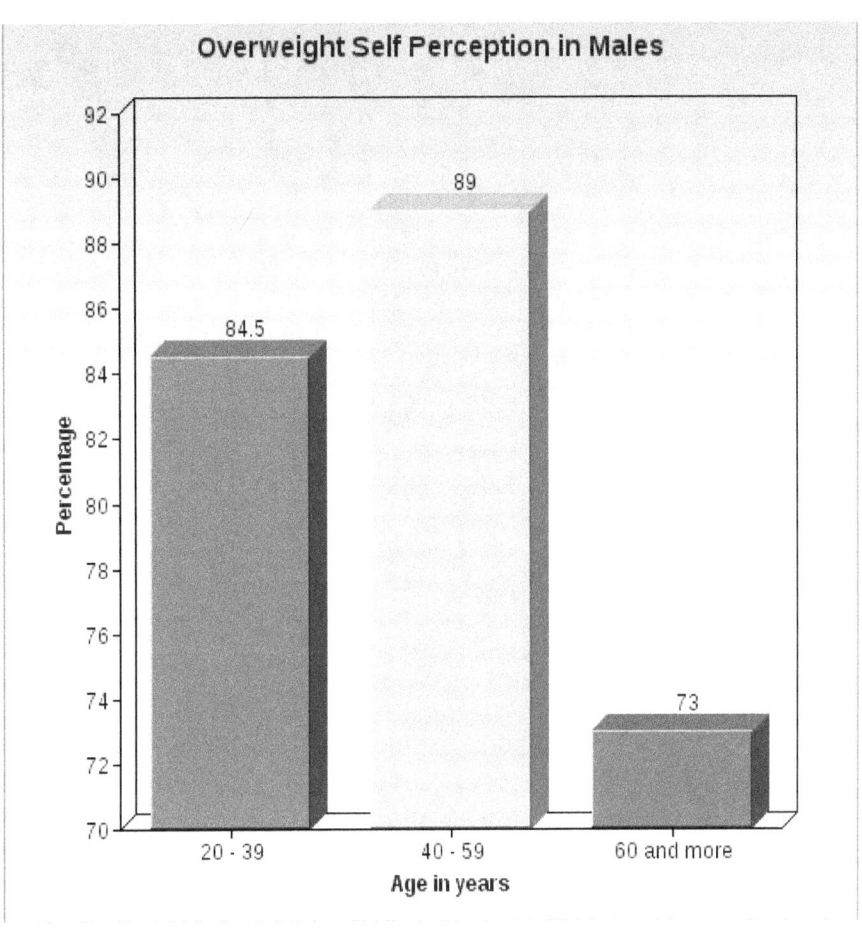

Similarly here's a graphical representation of the percentage of women who think they are overweight.

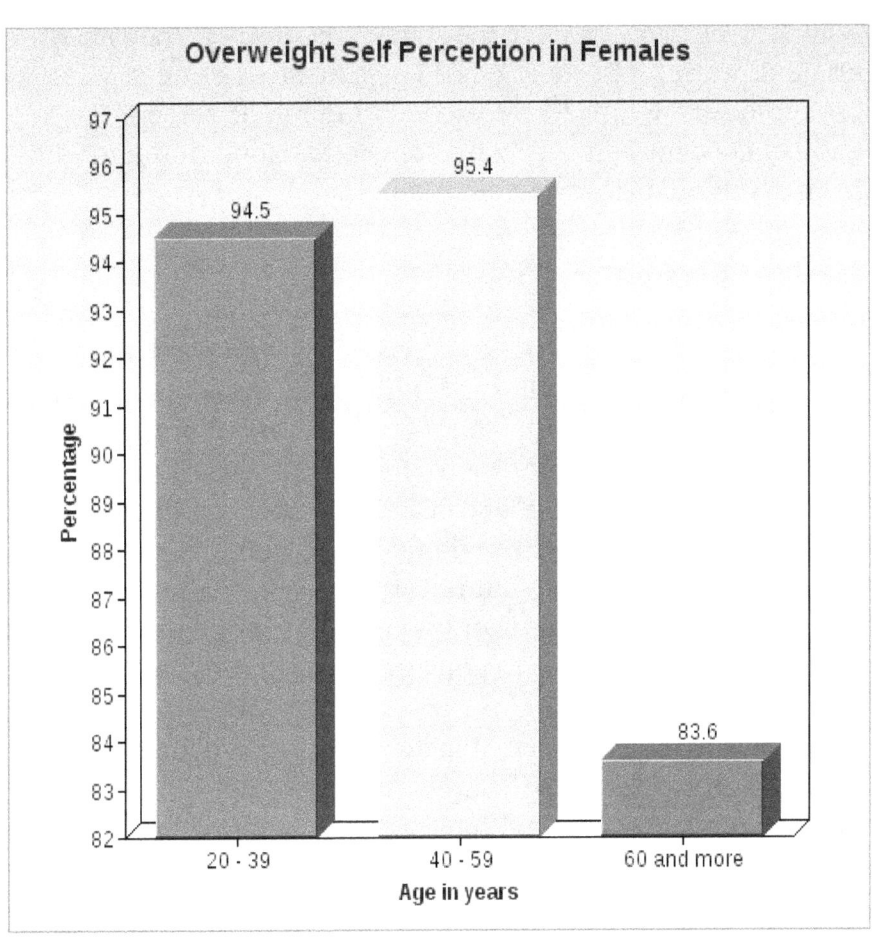

There is a need to protect yourself from erroneous beliefs and perceptions that you may tend to acquire with time, or when you move out on the streets and come across other people who may or may not have the shape you desire. When an on-line publication, Psychology Today, consulted some psychologists, who had researched human self perceptions and beliefs, they came up with some interesting findings that I have dwelt on, below:

1. What's My Motivation?

Most of us, when starting an exercise program, are already thinking of the end result, i.e., "I will be like this soon". "I will be like this" is alright, but "soon" is bound to put pressure on you. If you are fixated on "soon", then you are missing the vital intermediate steps that can actually take you there. You can jump to that end, with a giant leap. It would be great if your body could do that, but unfortunately it cannot. So, take it one step at a time. This is only possible through motivation. When you actually learn to appreciate your body, as it is currently, and understand what's good for your body and take steps to bring it into shape, it is then that you feel inspired to do so. This inspiration will stay with you and keep motivating you time and again till you have actually attained the shape you had visualized yourself in some time earlier.

2. What's In It To Celebrate?

Physical activities are always challenging. Once you are able to exercise with ease, you should congratulate yourself, on being able to do so. It is a simple act, but in your hurry to reach the target, you probably forget to do this simple thing. When you are doing so, you are acknowledging the distance you have already traveled.

You should take time to rejoice a little; this can help overcome the stress you faced during the journey.

3. I Can Manage Without Discipline...

Professional athletes are able to achieve high standards of excellence in their sports because they discipline themselves by constantly reminding themselves about what they have set out to do. They are often guided by able planners who monitor their activities. You may not have such help but you can still achieve the same standards of excellence as professional players.

To do this, you have to discipline yourself just like these players. Adjusting the standards should only be done when you find that you are limited in your stamina, or endurance levels. Excuses should not be allowed to creep in.

4. I Can't Win...

When you are surrounded by good looking people, you are bound to feel the urge to fit in. You try to exercise, but try as you might, you don't get the results you expected to see. You feel dejected. This is probably what most overweight people face.

You should understand that this is normal human nature and that such thoughts will come, no matter how hard you try to avoid them. The harder you try to fight it, the more pressure you end up putting on yourself. This creates additional stress. Learn to take it in your stride. Things are always going wrong somewhere. This is your body, but every body is different and reacts differently to various stimuli, such as exercise.

So what if you couldn't get it? Consider the two graphs above. All those people who considered themselves overweight would have, at a certain point of time, felt dejected. But most of them go on to recover from such thoughts and get themselves into good shape that makes them as attractive as others they envied, earlier. This is a cyclical process, and more and more people are trying to look good.

5. Am I Becoming My Own Enemy?

You may not believe or recognize this, but when you put yourself under undue pressure, you could possibly end up becoming your own biggest enemy, being a perfectionist, berating yourself on targets missed, cursing yourself, etc.

It is hard to identify these tendencies in yourself; probably someone close to you could point this out.

How Changing Your Thinking Can Effect Positive Change

That our thoughts govern our actions is well known. But how can this affect weight loss and the shape of your body, either positively or negatively?

A disturbed person suffers from stress, emotional upheaval and sorrow, or may even be overjoyed on some occasions. This stress results in the release of hormones in the blood stream that can affect the body's basal metabolic rate.

Continuous suffering from such stress could negate the effect of all your physical efforts to either lose or maintain weight. Such a prolonged state of mind where there are more negative emotions should be controlled, if necessary, with professional help. Otherwise, you will not see any benefits accruing from your physical efforts.

You may not be able to overcome your emotions, just by telling yourself so. As a first step, identify all the thoughts that you have had in the past few weeks or months when you have been exercising. Assess how much effort you have expended, physically, to get into shape and how much you have really benefited by it. Any mismatch would indicate that you have been losing, rather than winning. You might have felt an urge to stop exercising, or skip it, for a period of time. If such thoughts did arise, it's time to take corrective measures. The physical symptoms of such thoughts can be noticed when you tire easily, quicker than normal, or when you prefer to shorten your exercise routine, or tend to avoid certain muscle building exercises that require strength.

Acknowledging these self defeating thoughts might not be easy for you. Looking at and admiring something beautiful, or taking a walk in the park can help you overcome stress. Walking at a steady pace can force you to concentrate on maintaining the pace which will in turn help you concentrate on your aim which is getting a flat waist.

Sometimes undesired emotions can be overcome by a steady paced physical activity. Learn to bring your emotions under control through what ever you can comfortably do, and you will see better results with your exercise regime.

1. Overcoming The Need To Feel Appreciated

All of us, at certain points of time, feel the need to be appreciated for something or other. Likewise, when you are concentrating hard on weight loss and improving your looks, you will certainly want to be praised for your successes. This is human nature. We develop this psychology in childhood. But as we age, we tend to retain this in some degree. As an adult, now you have the ability to discern and choose the right path. Use this ability now to ask yourself, "Do I really need to be appreciated? How will that benefit me?" There is a feel good factor and it's satisfying to be praised. But you are also making yourself dependent on others' perceptions. That's a mistake. What if some people make an adverse remark about your looks? They may not know how hard you have worked to achieve this state. They may be comparing you with a different image that they have in their minds.

Block this out. It will take practice and require you to be patient. Overcoming this urge is important, along with relying on honest statistics that you have noted down. If you can block this, you are also protecting yourself from a stimulus for stress.

You are not working out to please others, but only your own self. You should perceive a good remark from others, as a bonus. Feedback is always good and necessary, but you should always depend on your own statistics.

2. Changing Focus

A lot of people will tell you to think positively. But how you do that is what most will not be able to answer. Though you can do it in many ways, it's better to adopt simple methods. You could check your weight and the waist size records, for instance. There will certainly be a difference, if not a marked difference. Take this as what you have achieved, with a lot of hard work. It was hard because you were not exercising earlier. But you are exercising now. Later on, when your body starts burning fat faster and your muscles become stronger, you won't have to work so hard to achieve your objective.

Failures are eye catching, and linger around longer. That also happens because of thinking selectively about negatives. But have you focused on what difference the exercises have made to your body. Touch, press and feel your abdomen. Do you feel the muscle getting stronger there? When you pull back your abdomen, how do you feel? How long can you hold it back? If you can feel the muscle now in your ab that you did not feel earlier, you have made progress.

Now, tell yourself, "If I continue this, later, I will feel it becoming stronger, day by day." This is not some kind of artificial consolation. This is to help progress onto the next state. Alternatively, can you twist around freely, and much more easily than before? If you can, that is a gain.

When you develop a rhythm for your exercise, your body gets comfortable with the pace of your exercise. You don't feel drained after each day of exercise. It becomes part of your life and easier to focus on just exercising when you want to exercise.

Below, I have given a graphical representation of the amount of time people devote to exercise. In a survey conducted by the American Time Use Survey group on people who are 15 years of age and above, it was noticed that people dedicate almost one hour for some form of exercise. It is clear that most people find it easy to integrate one hour of exercise into their daily lives even when they are busy. They are able to maintain this over a period of time only because they changed their focus -- from a muscular looking body, to more about getting into and staying in shape.
See the page here:
http://www.bls.gov/spotlight/2008/sports/data.htm#chart02

Here's the representation of the data, in a chart:

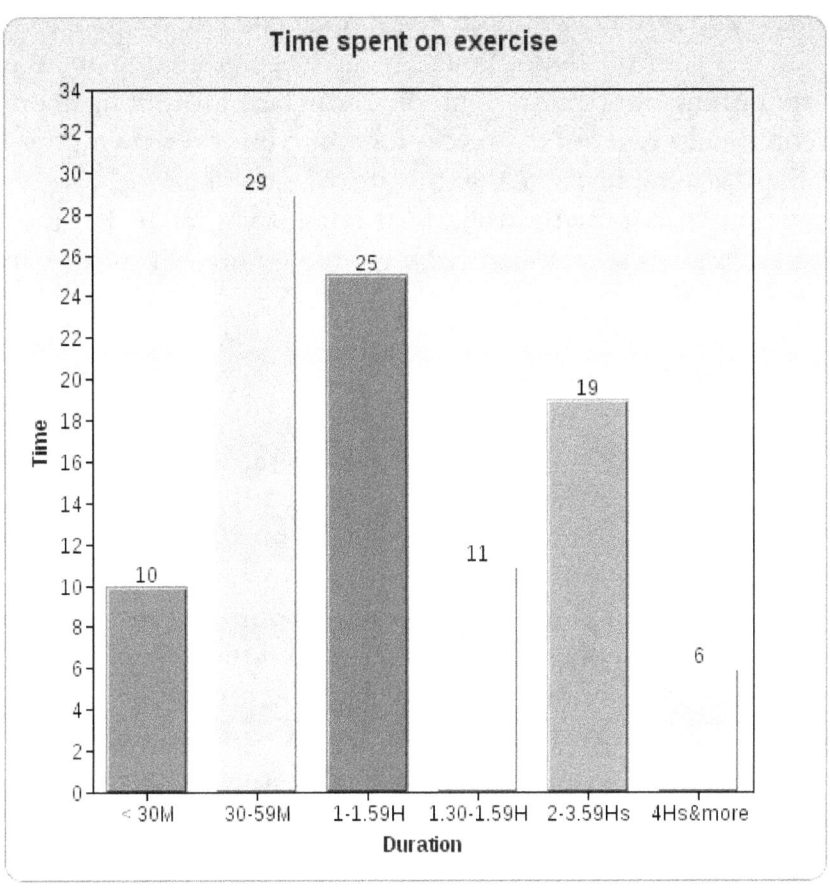

3. Have You Talked?

When you talk to somebody, you hear yourself talking and discussing what's on your mind. When you talk to the right person about how your body feels, he or she will be able to point out your mistakes. You may have been thinking about a certain thing but couldn't pinpoint how it fit in. Talking about it could help you put the pieces together. But even if you miss it, there is a high chance that the other person hearing you may point it out to you. Talking also helps you relax. But the need to relax is something that we often ignore. The next point points this out.

4. Learning To Relax

How many hours have you spent exercising, and how many have you spent relaxing your mind and body? You can relax, physically, by resting, stretching, etc., but how do you clear all those doubts that arise -- on their own -- in your mind -- time and again? If you are frequently asking yourself questions like, "Am I doing the right exercise the right way?" and "Am I doing enough to improve my looks?", you need to let go at some point or you will end up tired, confused and frustrated. The result will naturally be that you will want to give up everything, and relax. Almost every one of us has been through this stage at some time in our lives. This feeling is the same as the frustration you feel when you are trying too hard to get something, but end up falling back.

Learn to relax. If you can't complete your schedule today because you are simply too tired, then you can skip the rest. But do not let this tendency cloud your judgment using it as a cover for laziness.

Coping With Changes

The physical effort you have put in so far will have caused some change in your body's hormone levels. The hormonal secretions increase when you exercise. This is a physical response of your body to the strain you are applying on it. With regular exercise, you will learn to identify certain changes that occur when you exercise, as compared to otherwise. But there are also certain unnoticed changes that occur in your thought processes. If you are doing different tasks, all these are having an effect on your mind.

There is bound to be a level of anxiety and uncertainty in your mind which can be similar to the "fear of the unknown". Add to this your own expectations from yourself and you are developing a stage where you end up into an avoidable void.

Anticipate some changes in your body and your life as you exercise. Accept these changes as results of your effort. Physical changes are easily noticed and as these are favored are easily acceptable. But if you have to dedicate more time and are feeling frustrated, this state of mind has to be accepted just like normal physical changes to your body. The more you try to resist or refuse to accept changes the more pressure you are likely to be creating inside yourself.

- **Attitude**

Accepting changes requires an attitudinal change. How you view exercises, from now on, will decide how close to your goal you get. Your attitude determines what will be the outcome of your physical efforts, the same way with weight loss programs, as with other things.

For example, how willing are you to accept the suggestions I have made in this report? Even if you don't agree with me, you can try to put some of these suggestions into practice, and find out if all this is true, or just crap. Now, you are thinking. If you had had a strong adverse attitude to what is told by others you wouldn't have covered so much of what is written here.

An irritable and impatient person would have given up, by now. But the fact that you have followed through for so long, you have shown some willingness to learn, and possibly, to change. If you have been an easily frustrated person till now but have managed to come thus far, it reveals your attitude and self control. Now you just have to convert this attitude into physical actions that will help you change your body for the better.

Preventing Weight Gain, after Loss – (The body craves what it lacks!)

You will come across many people who'll tell you that they managed to reduce their weight significantly. But one look at them will convince you that this is not true. It's easy to believe that their giving in to hunger pangs after losing a whole lot of weight (and undoing all their hard work) is a sign of mental weakness in such people. This isn't true, either.
Most people who lose weight regain what they have lost and then some. These people have most likely been on a very restricted diet that did not provide balanced nutrition in all three areas: protein, carbohydrate, and fat.

There is a biological factor in both men and women behind regaining weight. After you've been denying your body certain nutrients for an extended period of time, your body literally *craves* that nutrient. Smoking 'pot' produces the same, but more dramatic reaction. It produces an immediate depletion of sugar in the brain – which results in wanting to eat every piece of candy in sight!

If you've been denying yourself fat, for example, after you take "that one odd bite which will do no harm because you have already reduced your weight by a lot," your body will actually compel you to eat more of it.

In fact, research conducted by Wing and Phelan (2005) on members of the National Weight Control Registry, found that people *do* give into strong eating urges once they have reduced their weight.
People suffering from depression were also susceptible to weight regain. The gain can be over 5 lbs. The findings also showed that those who were able to maintain a stable weight for a period of 2 years were likely to maintain their weight under control for longer periods, the risk of weight regain in such people was reduced by as much as 50%. You can read the complete report, here:
http://www.unm.edu/~lkravitz/Article%20folder/winning.html

The findings also support the belief that with care and a strong will people will be able to maintain their gained body shape for a long period in their lifetime. Personally, I take issue with this interpretation of the data. I believe that a balanced diet eaten consistently is much more important for maintaining weight loss than is a "strong will".

Another reason for weight regain is that people tend to reduce the vigorous physical activity that helped them lose the weight in the first place. It's true that once weight is reduced by a lot, you don't have to be so vigorous, subsequently. But reducing it to a bare minimum could undo all that you have managed to do till now.

Your motivation will slacken once you have reached your goal. You will notice this when you start slipping behind in your exercise schedule.

An experimental study conducted by some universities and medical centers in parts of Dakota, Carolina, Minnesota and New Jersey revealed that the weight regain percentage lay in the ranges between 5% to 30.6%. There was no appreciable change in the weight regain manner between men and women. More clear results of this experiment can be seen here:
http://www.nature.com/oby/journal/v11/n10/full/oby2003166a.html

More information regarding weight regain after loss is difficult to come by as there is limited research on this topic. There is also a feeling that most people who regain weight have not been able to reduce weight by much, but I don't think that feeling is accurate.

In an article published, and available at
http://www.ncbi.nlm.nih.gov/pmc/articles/PMC2679815/ , (a medical journal website), Robert Ross of Queens University of Kingston, Ont. claims that research by different groups about how people regain weight, after losing some weight, found that the participants managed to reduce their weight by almost 4 kgs, regained between 2.5 - 4.9 kgs to 4.0 - 5.5 kgs.

The studies also revealed that people who weighed themselves regularly as a means of keeping their weight under control, fared better, compared to people who did not. Another not-so-surprising result was that those who maintained their rate of physical activity were better able to maintain their weight than others. A controlled diet can also prevent gain in weight, once it has been reduced.

A publication of the American College of Sports Medicine, whose results can be seen at http://static.publico.clix.pt/docs/pesoemedida/Acsm_Positio n_Statement_Weight_Loss.pdf shows that participants who exercised for more than 280 minutes every week were able to maintain weight, whereas those who exercised for less than 200 minutes regained weight. The study also showed that an activity rate (maximum heart rate) of 55% to 69% is adequate to maintain weight in people who have lost weight. It also states that most people who have reduced their weight, if they avoid seeking professional help, regain all the weight they had lost within a period of 3 to 5 years.

Diet alone is not an effective strategy in maintaining weight loss. This report at the Medscape CME website, http://cme.medscape.com/viewarticle/558092?src=mp&spon= 17&uac=101ST , can be taken as an example. It states that in an analysis of the data gathered by the National Health and Nutritional Examination Survey (NHANES) during the period 1999 to 2002 on 1310 participants in the U.S.A, nearly 33.5% had regained lost weight by about 5%.

The website also carries a comment by Dr. Traci Mann, Ph.D. of the University of California in Los Angeles, about the regaining of weight by most people who relied on diets to reduce weight. This data included people from different race backgrounds living in the U.S.A. However a thing to note in this research is that the participants did not confirm their daily intake of calories.

An important point to be understood here is the importance of "triggers" or "medical triggers" as used by doctors concerned with behavioral medicine. Such doctors under the National Weight Control Registry (seen here - http://www.ajcn.org/cgi/content/full/82/1/222S) have noticed that people who started on a weight loss program due to medical triggers -- which could be as simple as a doctor telling his or her patient to lose weight, or alternatively, the death of a family member owing to weight related issues -- fared much better than those who were prompted by non medical triggers such as superficial looks. Such people who were prompted by medical triggers were more likely to maintain their weight and control weight regain.

Maintaining the Level of Reduced Weight

Once you have successfully managed to reduce your weight to the desired level, you still have to work to keep it in that state. The primary strategy that is applied to keep weight under check is regular physical activity. But even though all weight control experts agree on this point, they differ on the level of physical activity and the exercise needed to maintain the level of reduced weight.

The University of Virginia Health System, on its website, offers some tips to help those struggling to maintain their reduced weight. Although anybody who has has been successful in maintaining his/her weight for a few months, after reducing it, will consider these points as too general. I would, nevertheless, like to mention these for the benefit of those who are confused, and need some support.

The website recommends:

- Avoiding diets with extremely low content of calories that can alter the body's rate of metabolism. This will prevents your body from trying to recover lost weight later.

- Changing your life style and way of living (most experts recommend this, anyway).

- Keeping your weight loss target to a maximum of 2 pounds every week during the reduction period so that your body gets time to adjust to the change. A rapid change can signal a threat to the body which then tries to make up for the lost weight by increasing weight at the first opportunity.

- Like the participants at the National Weight Control Registry, here too, the university research findings recommend that those who want to maintain their state of reduced weight should continue to seek some kind of professional guidance even after weight reduction to prevent weight gain. Various reasons can be attributed for this particular requirement, one being that people who notice others who have also successfully reduced their weight may be influenced by their efforts and successes along with the advice of professionals.

- The same group under the NWCR also used a controlled intake of food (diet) to maintain their weight. But it is necessary to reach a level of balance. To do this, once you have hit the bottom of the weight scale, you can experiment by slowly increasing your calorie intake by 200 in healthy food for a period of a week. This increased level of calorie should not freeze or reverse the weight loss which should actually continue to decrease as you try. If your weight reduces despite this higher intake of calories, then you can add a further amount, in equal measure, till you attain a balance. This will require you to experiment over a period time. Once your weight stabilizes, you will have to freeze the level of calorie intake.

- The last tip, but by no means the least, is to keep up with a regular exercise schedule so that your body's functions are not disturbed in any way. After the desired level you need not continue with as strenuous exercises as before. Instead, you can slow down, somewhat, to a level of expending 1500 - 2000 calories every week.

In a study done by doctors at the National Weight Control Registry, it was noted that those who were prompted by medical reasons to lose weight also managed their post weight reduction maintenance better than those who did have a medical reason for weight loss. Such members regained 2 kgs lesser than those without a medical trigger to prompt them to lose weight.
(see here - http://www.ajcn.org/cgi/content/full/82/1/222S)

Relapsing And Subsequent Recovery

The NWCR study also includes a report on how some people who had regained weight following weight reduction, subsequently managed to reduce the regained weight.
http://www.ajcn.org/cgi/content/full/82/1/222S

The report also pointed out that only those who had regained about a kilo or two were the most likely to successfully lose the regained weight. As the regained weight increased, it was less likely that those participants would succeed in reducing their regained weight.

Here are some of the findings and suggestions put forth by the doctors monitoring weight loss and regain. These points, though simple, are an indication of how simple it is to regain weight and undo all your efforts at weight reduction. It also indicates how casual we can get.

-- Monitor your weight regularly. With such regular monitoring, you can get a better idea of how much you've lost as well as how much still needs to be done.

-- Exercise regularly, or use similar sports or other physical activity that burns body fat and lowers weight. Being active in this manner will keep your body's fat burning process working and you will lose stored fat. This will prevent storage of fat in your body.

-- Never skip breakfast. But this is what most of us do when hurrying to the office or when we feel too lazy to eat before rushing out the door. When you work with low energy intake, your body does everything to compensate for the missing intake, including storing fat. Over time, this becomes a regular feature, and your body tends to store more fat than it actually uses. Thus, avoiding breakfast has several consequences other than just making you feel tired. As more and more people understand the value of eating breakfast, they look for more ways of having breakfast -- at home or on the way to work. Its value is increasingly being recognized among the well educated adult population -- take a look at the statistical data provided at this website: http://www.mrbreakfast.com/glossary_term.asp?glossaryID= 152)

-- Eat a controlled diet with measured intake of calories. Like the physical activity, which has to be constant and regular, so should be the food items you eat. A proper balance can be maintained by noting down what you eat, comparing it with a food chart to identify how many calories you are ingesting, and then tailoring your exercise program accordingly.

-- Observe any abnormal growth in weight and immediately change your schedule of exercise for a few days till that abnormality is countered.

If you want to know how many people actually follow these suggestions, and how successful they are then look at the statistics provided here: http://www.nwcr.ws/Research/default.htm

The following are some of the statistics mentioned on the page:

- 90% of their participants used one hour of exercise per day (i.e. increased physical activity) as a means of preventing weight regain.
- 78% of the participants ate their breakfast to prevent any untoward regain in weight . . . This after realizing the benefits of eating breakfast.
- 62% of the participants spent less hours watching TV. This time period could have been higher earlier.
- 75% of the participants reported weighing themselves regularly to keep tabs on their weight.

Returning to Gary Pierce, referred to at the beginning of this report, he was not only able to reduce weight significantly, he successfully kept his weight under check. If you want to see an older example of how people have successfully checked weight regain, take a look at the example of Drew Saur here: http://www.nwcr.ws/stories.htm. Drew has traveled a great distance, since his overweight days. He wants to share his experiences for the benefit of others who can be inspired by his achievements to stay thin, fit and good looking.

Or look at another example, that of Michal Eakin, who, once she lost weight, prioritized maintaining her condition and has been able to do so by her sheer determination. Or better still, take the example of Charles Aloisio, who, to quote him, discusses his "relationship with food". He resolved to perfect his regime and gain control over his body. His first victory was in shedding almost 100 pounds of unnecessary weight from his body. His next task was to stay that way. Today, to his credit, he has recorded a timespan, spread over 16 years, as a period of controlled weight without much fluctuation.

Such success stories are worthy of awe. If you really want to know how close you can get to these successful people, I suggest you take a photo of yourself when you are overweight or obese. After a few months, when your old clothes are way to big for you, take a look at your photo that you took before, and then compare it with your reflection in the mirror. More than the flat tummy, it is the feeling of triumph that comes with it that's your best reward!

Epilogue

When Jim's airline fired him from his job, and then, Jenny lost hers, it was the turning point of their lives.

Jim had to settle for a bar-tending job, at a local club. Jenny got another job, and though it didn't pay as much, as her previous one, life, for the couple, began to get better.

And then, Jim bumped into his old boss at the airline, who offered Jim his old job back if he could get into shape, and fast. Jim resolved to eat sensibly and shed weight...

He was really keen to get back to his old airline - sporting a flat tummy, and looking sexy.
And he did.

These days, when someone compliments Jim, and says, "Hey Jim, you look great!" Jim knows he's back on track. When he was sacked from his airline job, Jim chose to use it as a wake-up call when he could easily have gone to pieces.

It all boiled down to motivation – from within. Jim's positive frame of mind meant that Jenny and Jim were both gainers in the end.

Jenny and Jim are finally ready to start a family - in fact, Jenny is expecting their first child!

TAKE-AWAYS

1. The body craves what it lack. This is the major reason why diets that rely on restricting one of the major macro-nutrients – protein, carbohydrate, fat – absolutely do not work for the long term. To lose weight and keep it off, a balanced diet is essential.

2. The body craves what it lacks – 2. This is also a major reason why people who primarily eat foods that are refined and/or highly processed (those with no or low natural micro-nutrients – vitamins, minerals, etc. – may need to eat more total food which tends to be stored as fat than someone eating healthier, more natural micro-nutrient rich foods.

3. Will power is a very poor tool for long-term success. Will power by its very nature is the act of fighting your natural impulses. This uses up a lot of energy. At some point, you'll get tired of using your energy this way – and stop. Then all of your hard work will have been for nothing because whatever changes you've made will revert to their former condition.

4. Prepare your mind for success and your body will follow. Learn how to get out of your own way. To this end, I'm recommending the following book: The Secret Code of Success by Noah St. John, c. 2009.

5. Deciding to change how you look must be a personal decision for personal reasons. However, being successful in that decision is made easier with support and help from others rather than trying to go it alone. This includes support groups, family, friends, a personal trainer, gym membership, or some other kind of professional help.

6. As with most things, the difference between success and failure is in the details. Pay Attention To The **DETAILS!**

7. This one's a no-brainer: *the exercises and diet recommendations won't work if you don't actively put them to use.* The exercises, if done regularly with proper technique, will work. If you eat healthier food with sufficient natural micro-nutrients, you will have better muscle tone and more energy. Enough said. . .

References

American Obesity Association's fact sheet about obesity in the USA:
http://obesity1.tempdomainname.com/subs/fastfacts/obesity_US.shtml

National Institute of Diabetes and Digestive and Kidney Diseases (NIDDK) perspective on obesity in adults on the Wrong Diagnosis webpage:
http://www.wrongdiagnosis.com/artic/understanding_adult_obesity_niddk.htm

A Wrong Diagnosis view of obesity and its prevalence in American adults:
- http://www.wrongdiagnosis.com/o/obesity/basics.htm

Some participants who have successfully reduced weight registered with the National Weight Control Registry:
http://www.nwcr.ws/stories.htm

A real life success story of a participant under the National Weight Control Registry: http://www.nwcr.ws/stories.htm

Statistics from Google regarding gym usage and membership, church and rehabilitation among American adults:
http://answers.google.com/answers/threadview/id/138544.html

Facts and figures about time management presented by Dr. Donald E. Wetmore of Productivity Institute:
http://www.dovico.com/time-management-factsandfigures.html

Results of evaluations on gyms and fitness centers:
http://www.healthandfitness.com/resources/gym_evaluation
.asp

A list of excuses often used by people as complied by the
International Health Racquet and Sportsclub Association a
non profit organization:
http://cms.ihrsa.org/index.cfm?fuseaction=page.viewPage&p
ageID=20876

How the Journal of American Medical Association uses the
power of Internet for improvement public health and
behavior: http://jama.ama-
assn.org/cgi/content/abstract/285/9/1172

Food and Drug Administration report on the money spent on
health improvement:
http://www.worldometers.info/weight-loss/

Data from the Bureau of Labor Statistics of the United States
Department of Labor:
http://www.bls.gov/spotlight/2008/sports/data.htm#chart02

Data from the Center for Disease Control given on the Medical
News website: http://www.news-
medical.net/news/20090904/Americans-health-perceptions-
contradict-national-statistics.aspx

Statistics about physical activity given by National Institute of
Diabetes and Digestive and Kidney Diseases (NIDDK):
http://www.win.niddk.nih.gov/statistics/index.htm#other

Self perception in men and women about being overweight on
the Infoplease website:
http://www.infoplease.com/ipa/A0763634.html

Data about exercise and sports among men women and teenagers:
http://www.bls.gov/spotlight/2008/sports/data.htm#chart02

An article by Len Kravitz, Ph.D. about the "Secrets of Long-Term Weight Loss":
http://www.unm.edu/~lkravitz/Article%20folder/winning.html

Results of research about the "Impact of weight loss and regain on the quality of life":
http://www.nature.com/oby/journal/v11/n10/full/oby2003166a.html

Research results and findings about weight regain by Robert Ross, Ph.D. CMAJ.JAMC journal website:
http://www.ncbi.nlm.nih.gov/pmc/articles/PMC2679815/

Weight loss and regain prevention strategies form the American College of Sports Medicine:
http://static.publico.clix.pt/docs/pesoemedida/Acsm_Position_Statement_Weight_Loss.pdf

Research and findings about dieting and weight loss on the Medscape CME website:
http://cme.medscape.com/viewarticle/558092?src=mp&spon=17&uac=101ST

An article about maintaining reduced weight over a long period by Rena R Wing and Suzanne Phelan published by The American Journal of Clinical Nutrition:
http://www.ajcn.org/cgi/content/full/82/1/222S

Statistics and latest trends about breakfast consumed:
http://www.mrbreakfast.com/glossary_term.asp?glossaryID=
152

Facts and statistics from National Weight Control Registry regarding weight loss and its methods:
http://www.nwcr.ws/Research/default.htm

Successful participants who have managed to reduce weight under the National Weight Control Registry:
http://www.nwcr.ws/stories.htm

About the Author

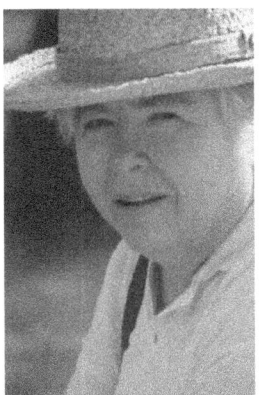

Joyce Zborower graduated from Bradley University, Peoria, Illinois, in 1965 with a B.S. degree and in 1969 with an M.A., both in clinical psychology. She worked for several years as a school psychologist in South Chicago before moving to Arizona in 1975 to become a full-time mom to her two little girls. She still lives in Arizona.

Books by Joyce Zborower

My Amazon page: http://amzn.to/MIKKpJ
The Trust – a cautionary tale
Little Mysteries – a short story
Handcrafted Jewelry Step by Step – beginner and intermediate original designs
Handcrafted Jewelry Photo Gallery – cast jewelry -- fabricated jewelry
Wire Jewelry Photo Gallery – Original Designs
Creations in Wood Photo Gallery – jewelry boxes, screens, storage ideas
Bargello Quilts Photo Gallery – quilt wall hangings
Bargello Train Quilt – cutting and sewing instructions
Sell Your Work – how to turn your craft into your business
Psychology of Success – how to have success when trying to change how you look
No Work Vegetable Gardening – for in-ground, raised beds, or container gardening
How To Eat Healthy – foods to eat . . . foods to avoid
The Truth About Olive Oil – benefits, curing methods, remedies

Paperback Books

Psychology of Success – how to succeed when trying to change how you look
No Work Vegetable Gardening – for in-ground, raised beds, or container gardening
The Truth About Olive Oil – benefits, curing methods, remedies
Sell Your Work – how to turn your craft into your business
Little Mysteries – a short story

Español Libros (Spanish language Books) – Available or Coming Soon

Mi página de Amazon http://amzn.to/MlKKpJ
El Fideicomiso – fábula con moraleja
Pequeños Misterios– cuento
Joyas Hechas a Mano Paso a Paso – diseños originales para nivel principiantes e intermedio
Joyas Hechas a Mano - Galería de fotos – joyas fundidas— joyas forjadas
Joyas de Alambre - Galería de fotos – Diseños originales
Creaciones en Madera- Galería de fotos – joyeros, biombos, ideas de almacenaje
Quilts Tipo Bargello- Galería de fotos – tapices de quilt
Quilt de Tren en Bargello– instrucciones para cortar y coser
Venda su Trabajo – como transformar tu arte en negocio
La Psicología del Éxito – cómo tener éxito al tratar de cambiar tu apariencia
Huerto sin Esfuerzo – para jardinería en el suelo, elevada o en contenedor
Como Comer Sano – comidas para comer…comidas para evitar
La Verdad Acerca del Aceite de Oliva– beneficios, métodos de curación, remedios

Other Recommended Books

The Confession of a Trust Magnate ----- by George Allen Yuille

Picture the combined navies of the world anchored off our seaboard cities, the

combined armies of the world in possession
of our inland cities, envoys from each
nation congregated at Washington
partitioning our country, the entire population
being apportioned as slaves to do the bidding
of the conquerors.
Would you be interested?
An equally appalling situation confronts
the people of this country today.
Read of it in the pages of this book.

This book was written in 1911. It's message is critical for today – 2012.

Questions and Comments

I'd love to hear your thoughts.
Email me at admin@hunting4clients.com

Need help?

Are you an aspiring writer who's having trouble getting your book published? My company does book editing and formatting and posts client's books to Create Space, Smashwords, and KDP.

My GURANTEE: Your book will pass the Smashwords' Meat-grinder and Auto-vetter and/or the formatting requirements of Create Space and/or KDP or you pay nothing.

You can reach me at admin@hunting4clients.com

One Last Thing Before You Go. . .

If you believe the book is worth sharing, would you take a few seconds and let your friends know about it? If it turns out to make a difference in their lives, they'll be forever grateful to you. As will I.

All the best
Joyce Zborower

or go to my Amazon page: http://amzn.to/MIKKpJ and click the book cover to get to the 'Review This Book' button.